Youthful You
Ageless Adventures for Active Aging

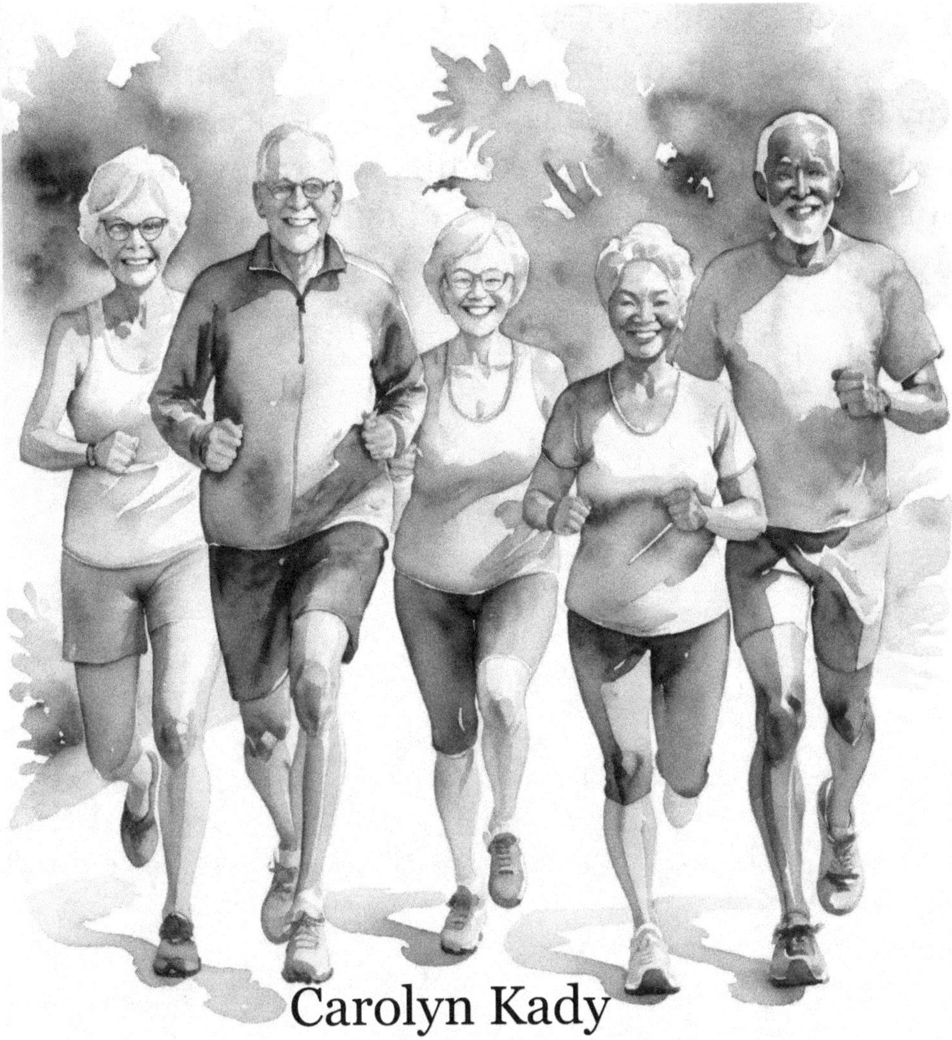

Carolyn Kady

Published by Carolyn Kady

Legal Disclaimer:

The information provided in this book is for general informational and educational purposes only. It is not intended as legal, medical, financial, or other professional advice. The author and publisher of this ebook are not engaged in rendering legal, medical, financial, or other professional services.

Table of Contents

Chapter 1: The Benefits of Active Aging In this chapter, we will explore the numerous benefits of staying active as we age. From improved physical health to enhanced mental well-being, active aging can help us live longer, happier, and more fulfilling lives. Pg. 1

Chapter 2: Setting Goals for Physical Activity Setting goals for physical activity is essential for maintaining an active lifestyle. In this chapter, we will discuss the importance of goal-setting and provide tips for creating realistic and achievable goals that will keep you motivated and engaged. Pg. 5

Chapter 3: Finding the Right Exercise Routine Finding the right exercise routine is key to staying active and healthy as we age. In this chapter, we will explore different types of exercise and help you identify the best routine for your needs and goals. Pg. 10

Chapter 4: Nutrition Tips for Active Aging Proper nutrition plays a crucial role in active aging. In this chapter, we will provide tips for eating a healthy diet that will support your physical activity and overall well-being. Pg. 15

Chapter 5: Mental Health and Active Aging Mental health is just as important as physical health when it comes to active aging. In this chapter, we will discuss strategies for maintaining a healthy mindset and coping with the challenges that come with aging. Pg. 20

Chapter 6: Social Connections and Community Involvement Social connections and community involvement are vital for staying active and engaged as we age. In this chapter, we will explore the benefits of staying connected with others and provide tips for building and maintaining meaningful relationships. Pg. 25

Chapter 7: The Importance of Sleep for Active Aging Quality sleep is essential for overall health and well-being, especially as we age. In this chapter, we will discuss the importance of sleep and provide tips for improving your sleep habits. Pg. 29

Chapter 8: Preventing and Managing Chronic Conditions Chronic conditions can present challenges to active aging, but with the right strategies, they can be managed effectively. In this chapter, we will discuss ways to prevent and manage chronic conditions to support your active lifestyle. Pg. 34

Chapter 9: Balancing Work and Leisure in Retirement Retirement can provide opportunities for new adventures and experiences, but it also comes with its own set of challenges. In this chapter, we will discuss strategies for balancing work and leisure in retirement to ensure a fulfilling and active lifestyle. Pg. 39

Chapter 10: Embracing Technology for Active Aging Technology can be a valuable tool for staying active and connected as we age. In this chapter, we will explore ways to embrace technology to enhance your active aging journey. Pg. 44

Chapter 11: Travel and Adventure in Later Life Travel and adventure can add excitement and joy to later life. In this chapter, we will discuss the benefits of travel and provide tips for planning and enjoying adventures as you age. Pg. 48

Chapter 12: Cultivating a Positive Mindset A positive mindset is key to successful active aging. In this chapter, we will discuss strategies for cultivating a positive outlook and maintaining a sense of optimism as you navigate the challenges of aging. Pg. 52

Conclusion: Your Youthful You Journey In conclusion, active aging is a journey that requires dedication, commitment, and a positive mindset. By incorporating the strategies and tips provided in this book, you can embark on your own Youthful You journey and enjoy a fulfilling and active lifestyle as you age. Pg. 56

Next Steps: Resources for Continued Active Aging To support your active aging journey, we have compiled a list of resources that can help you continue to stay active, healthy, and engaged. From fitness programs to mental health resources, these resources will provide you with the tools you need to thrive in your later years. Pg. 59

Chapter 1: The Benefits of Active Aging

As we continue to advance in age, the importance of maintaining an active and healthy lifestyle becomes increasingly apparent. The concept of active aging has gained significant traction in recent years, as more and more individuals seek ways to enhance their longevity and improve their quality of life. In this chapter, we will explore the benefits of active aging, including its impact on overall health, cognitive function, and social well-being.

Active aging encompasses a holistic approach to aging that focuses on staying physically, mentally, and socially engaged throughout the later years of life. This concept recognizes that aging is a natural and inevitable process, but also emphasizes that there are steps that individuals can take to promote healthy aging and enhance their well-being.

One of the key benefits of active aging is its positive impact on physical health. Regular exercise and physical activity have been shown to improve cardiovascular health, strengthen muscles and bones, and reduce the risk of chronic diseases such as diabetes and hypertension. By staying active, older adults can maintain their independence and mobility, allowing them to continue engaging in the activities they enjoy and living life to the fullest.

In addition to physical health, active aging also plays a crucial role in maintaining cognitive function and mental well-being. Studies have shown that engaging in mentally stimulating activities, such as reading, puzzles, and social interactions, can help preserve cognitive function and reduce the risk of cognitive decline. By challenging the mind and staying mentally active, older adults can enhance their memory, problem-solving skills, and overall cognitive abilities.

Furthermore, active aging promotes social well-being by encouraging older adults to stay connected with others and engage in meaningful relationships and activities. Social isolation is a common issue among older adults, particularly as they retire and lose regular contact with colleagues and friends. By participating in social activities, volunteering, and joining community groups, older adults can build a strong social support network and maintain a sense of purpose and belonging.

Overall, the benefits of active aging are numerous and wide-ranging, impacting not only individual health and well-being but also society as a whole. By promoting active aging, we can reduce healthcare costs, improve the quality of life for older adults, and create a more inclusive and age-friendly society.

In the following chapters, we will delve deeper into the specific components of active aging, including exercise, nutrition, mental health, and social engagement. We will explore practical strategies and tips for incorporating active aging into your daily life and discuss the potential challenges and barriers that may arise along the way.

In conclusion, active aging is a dynamic and empowering approach to aging that emphasizes the importance of staying physically, mentally, and socially engaged as we grow older. By embracing the principles of active aging, individuals can enhance their longevity, improve their quality of life, and age with vitality and grace. Join us on this journey towards healthier and happier aging, and discover the transformative power of active aging.

Chapter 2: Setting Goals for Physical Activity

Physical activity is essential for maintaining health and well-being, especially as we age. However, in order to reap the full benefits of exercise, it is important to set realistic and achievable goals. Setting goals can help you stay motivated, track your progress, and ensure that you are making the most of your physical activity routine. In this chapter, we will discuss how to create effective goals for active aging.

Assess Your Current Fitness Level

Before setting any goals, it is important to assess your current fitness level. This will help you determine where you are starting from and what areas you may need to focus on. You can assess your fitness level by taking a simple fitness test, such as a walking test or a flexibility test. You can also consult with a healthcare provider or a fitness professional for a more comprehensive evaluation.

Consider Your Health and Physical Limitations

When setting goals for physical activity, it is important to consider your health and physical limitations. If you have any medical conditions or physical limitations, it is crucial to take them into account when setting goals. Be sure to consult with your healthcare provider before starting any new exercise routine, especially if you have a chronic condition or are recovering from an injury.

Set Specific and Measurable Goals

When setting goals for physical activity, it is important to make them specific and measurable. Rather than setting a vague goal such as "I want to get in shape," try setting a more specific goal such as "I want to walk for 30 minutes five days a week." Setting measurable goals will help you track your progress and stay motivated.

Make Your Goals Realistic and Achievable

While it is important to challenge yourself, it is also important to make your goals realistic and achievable. Setting goals that are too ambitious can lead to frustration and burnout. Start with small, achievable goals and gradually increase the intensity or duration of your workouts as you progress. Remember, it's better to start small and build on your success than to set yourself up for failure.

Create a Plan

Once you have set your goals, it is time to create a plan to achieve them. This plan should include details such as what types of exercises you will do, how often you will exercise, and how you will track your progress. Be sure to include a mix of cardiovascular, strength training, and flexibility exercises in your plan to ensure a well-rounded workout routine.

Stay Consistent

Consistency is key when it comes to achieving your physical activity goals. Make a commitment to yourself to stick to your exercise plan, even on days when you may not feel motivated. Remember that progress takes time, and staying consistent with your workouts will help you reach your goals faster.

Track Your Progress

Tracking your progress is an important part of achieving your physical activity goals. Keep a journal or use a fitness app to record your workouts, track your progress, and celebrate your successes. Seeing how far you have come can be a great motivator to keep pushing forward.

Adjust Your Goals as Needed

As you progress in your fitness journey, it is important to periodically reassess your goals and make any necessary adjustments.

You may find that you need to increase the intensity of your workouts, set new goals, or change your exercise routine altogether. Be open to change and continue to challenge yourself to reach new heights.

Setting goals for physical activity is an important part of active aging. By creating realistic and achievable goals, making a plan, staying consistent, and tracking your progress, you can improve your health and well-being as you age. Remember, it's never too late to start reaping the benefits of regular exercise. So lace up your sneakers, set some goals, and get moving!

Chapter 3: Finding the Right Exercise Routine

When it comes to starting an exercise routine, one of the most important factors to consider is finding the right workout that suits your age and fitness level. With so many different types of exercises available, it can be overwhelming to choose the one that will help you reach your fitness goals while also being safe and effective. In this chapter, we will provide you with tips on how to select the best workouts for your individual needs.

Assess Your Current Fitness Level

Before choosing an exercise routine, it is essential to assess your current fitness level. This will help you determine which types of workouts are appropriate for you and which may be too challenging. Take into consideration factors such as your strength, flexibility, endurance, and any existing injuries or health conditions. If you are unsure about your fitness level, consider consulting with a fitness professional or your healthcare provider for guidance.

Consider Your Age

Age is an important factor to consider when selecting an exercise routine. As we age, our bodies may not be able to handle the same types of workouts that we were able to do in our younger years. It is crucial to choose exercises that are age-appropriate and take into account any age-related limitations or health concerns. For example, older adults may benefit from low-impact exercises such as walking, swimming, or yoga, while younger individuals may be able to handle more high-intensity activities like running or weightlifting.

Set Realistic Goals

Before starting an exercise routine, it is important to set realistic goals for yourself. Determine what you want to achieve with your workouts, whether it be weight loss, muscle gain, improved cardiovascular health, or increased flexibility.

Setting specific, measurable goals will help keep you motivated and focused as you work towards improving your fitness level.
Be sure to also consider your age and current fitness level when setting these goals to ensure they are attainable.

Choose a Variety of Workouts

To keep your exercise routine exciting and prevent boredom, it is beneficial to choose a variety of workouts that target different muscle groups and fitness goals. Incorporating a mix of cardiovascular exercises, strength training, and flexibility exercises will help you achieve a well-rounded fitness regimen. Consider trying different types of workouts such as cycling, Pilates, bodyweight exercises, or dance classes to keep your routine fresh and engaging.

Listen to Your Body

One of the most important tips for finding the right exercise routine is to listen to your body. Pay attention to how your body feels during and after exercise and adjust your workouts accordingly. If you experience pain or discomfort, stop the exercise and consult with a healthcare provider to determine the cause.
Pushing through pain can lead to injury and setbacks in your fitness journey. Remember that exercise should make you feel energized and invigorated, not exhausted and in pain.

Consult with a Fitness Professional

If you are unsure about which exercise routine is best for you, consider consulting with a fitness professional such as a personal trainer or exercise physiologist. These professionals can assess your fitness level, goals, and any limitations you may have, and create a tailored workout plan that is safe and effective for you.

They can also provide guidance on proper form, technique, and progression to help you reach your fitness goals efficiently.

In conclusion, finding the right exercise routine is essential for achieving your fitness goals and maintaining a healthy lifestyle.

By assessing your current fitness level, considering your age, setting realistic goals, choosing a variety of workouts, listening to your body, and consulting with a fitness professional, you can create a workout plan that is safe, effective, and enjoyable for you. Remember that consistency is key when it comes to exercise, so stay committed to your routine and be patient as you work towards improving your fitness level.

Chapter 4: Nutrition Tips for Active Aging

As we age, it is crucial to pay close attention to our nutrition in order to support an active and healthy lifestyle. A well-balanced diet can help older adults maintain their strength, energy levels, and overall well-being. In this chapter, we will discuss some important nutrition tips for active aging to help you stay healthy and vibrant as you grow older.

Eat a Variety of Nutrient-Dense Foods

One of the most important nutrition tips for active aging is to eat a variety of nutrient-dense foods. As we age, our bodies require fewer calories, but still need the same amount of nutrients, if not more. It is important to focus on foods that are rich in vitamins, minerals, fiber, and antioxidants. Some examples of nutrient-dense foods include fruits, vegetables, whole grains, lean proteins, and healthy fats. Aim to include a wide range of colors and flavors in your meals to ensure you are getting a variety of nutrients.

Stay Hydrated

Staying hydrated is essential for maintaining good health at any age, but it becomes even more important as we get older. Dehydration can lead to a variety of health issues, including fatigue, dizziness, and constipation. Aim to drink at least eight glasses of water per day, and more if you are active or live in a hot climate. You can also stay hydrated by consuming foods with high water content, such as fruits and vegetables.

Focus on Protein-Rich Foods

Protein is essential for maintaining muscle mass, strength, and overall health as we age. Older adults may require more protein than younger adults to support muscle maintenance and repair. Include a source of protein in each meal, such as lean meats, poultry, fish, eggs, dairy products, legumes, nuts, and seeds. Aim to spread your protein intake throughout the day to support optimal muscle function.

Limit Added Sugars and Salt

As we age, our bodies become more sensitive to the effects of added sugars and salt. Consuming too much sugar can increase the risk of obesity, diabetes, and heart disease, while excessive salt intake can lead to high blood pressure and other health issues. Limit your consumption of sugary beverages, sweets, baked goods, and processed foods high in salt. Instead, focus on whole, unprocessed foods that are naturally low in sugar and salt.

Include Fiber-Rich Foods

Fiber is important for digestive health, heart health, and weight management. As we age, it is common for digestive issues such as constipation to become more prevalent. Including fiber-rich foods in your diet can help prevent constipation and promote overall digestive health. Some good sources of fiber include fruits, vegetables, whole grains, legumes, nuts, and seeds. Aim to include a variety of high-fiber foods in your meals and snacks.

Consider Nutritional Supplements

In some cases, older adults may benefit from taking nutritional supplements to fill in any nutritional gaps in their diet. Talk to your healthcare provider before taking any supplements to ensure they are safe and appropriate for you. Some common supplements that may be beneficial for older adults include vitamin D, calcium, B vitamins, and omega-3 fatty acids. Remember, supplements should not replace a healthy diet but can be used to complement it.

Practice Mindful Eating

Mindful eating involves paying attention to your food choices, hunger cues, and eating habits. This can help you make healthier food choices, prevent overeating, and improve digestion.

Take the time to savor your meals, chew your food slowly, and listen to your body's hunger and fullness signals. Avoid distractions while eating, such as watching TV or using electronic devices, as this can lead to mindless eating and overconsumption.

By following these nutrition tips for active aging, you can support your health, vitality, and well-being as you grow older. Remember to consult with a healthcare provider or registered dietitian before making any major changes to your diet, especially if you have any underlying health conditions or dietary restrictions. With a balanced and nutrient-rich diet, you can stay active, vibrant, and healthy well into your golden years.

Chapter 5: Mental Health and Active Aging

As individuals age, it is essential to prioritize both physical and mental health to maintain overall well-being and quality of life. Mental health plays a critical role in active aging, influencing cognitive function, emotional well-being, and overall health outcomes. In this chapter, we will explore strategies for maintaining cognitive health and emotional well-being, ultimately promoting a fulfilling and vibrant lifestyle as we age.

Cognitive Health:

Cognitive health refers to the ability to think, learn, and remember. As we age, cognitive decline can occur, impacting memory, attention, and decision-making abilities. However, there are various strategies individuals can implement to maintain and even improve cognitive health as they age.

Stay Mentally Active: Engaging in mentally stimulating activities, such as puzzles, reading, and learning new skills, can help maintain cognitive function. Activities that challenge the brain, such as crossword puzzles or learning a new language, can promote mental agility and improve memory.

Stay Socially Engaged: Social interactions are essential for cognitive health. Engaging in social activities, such as joining clubs, volunteering, or participating in group outings, can help maintain cognitive function and reduce feelings of isolation.

Stay Physically Active: Physical exercise not only benefits physical health but also plays a crucial role in cognitive function. Regular exercise has been shown to improve memory, attention, and executive function. Aim for at least 30 minutes of moderate-intensity exercise most days of the week.

Maintain a Healthy Diet: A nutritious diet rich in fruits, vegetables, whole grains, and lean proteins can support cognitive function. Certain nutrients, such as omega-3 fatty acids found in fish, have been shown to benefit brain health. Limiting processed foods and sugar can also help maintain cognitive health.

Emotional Well-Being:

Emotional well-being refers to our overall emotional state and ability to cope with stress and challenges. As we age, emotional well-being can be influenced by various factors, including changes in health, relationships, and life circumstances. It is essential to prioritize emotional well-being to maintain a positive outlook and overall quality of life.

Practice Mindfulness: Mindfulness involves focusing on the present moment and accepting it without judgment.

Mindfulness practices, such as meditation or deep breathing exercises, can help reduce stress, anxiety, and negative emotions. Incorporating mindfulness into daily routines can promote emotional well-being.

Seek Support: Building strong social connections and seeking support from friends, family, or mental health professionals can enhance emotional well-being. Sharing feelings and experiences with others can provide comfort and validation, reducing feelings of loneliness and isolation.

Engage in Meaningful Activities: Participating in activities that bring joy, purpose, and fulfillment can improve emotional well-being. Whether it's pursuing a hobby, volunteering, or spending time with loved ones, engaging in activities that hold personal significance can boost mood and overall well-being.

Practice Self-Care: Taking care of oneself is essential for emotional well-being. Prioritizing self-care activities, such as getting enough sleep, eating well, and engaging in relaxation techniques, can help manage stress and promote emotional resilience.

In conclusion, mental health plays a vital role in active aging, influencing cognitive function, emotional well-being, and overall quality of life. By implementing strategies to maintain cognitive health and emotional well-being, individuals can promote a fulfilling and vibrant lifestyle as they age. Prioritizing mental health is essential for aging well and enjoying a meaningful and fulfilling life.

As we age, it can be easy to become more isolated and disconnected from the world around us. The demands of daily life, changes in health or mobility, and the loss of loved ones can all contribute to feelings of loneliness and social isolation. However, maintaining social connections and staying engaged in our communities is vital for our overall well-being and quality of life as we age.

Social connections play a crucial role in our mental and emotional health. Research has shown that individuals who have strong social networks are less likely to experience depression, anxiety, and cognitive decline as they age. Having regular social interactions can also help to reduce feelings of loneliness and isolation, and provide a sense of purpose and belonging.

Community involvement is another key aspect of healthy aging. By participating in activities and events in our communities, we can stay active, engaged, and connected to others. Whether it's volunteering at a local charity, joining a social club, or attending community events, being involved in our communities can provide a sense of fulfillment and connection to the world around us.

There are many ways to stay connected and involved as we age. Here are some tips for maintaining social connections and community involvement:

Stay in touch with family and friends: Make an effort to regularly reach out to loved ones, whether it's through phone calls, video chats, or in-person visits. Maintaining close relationships with family and friends can provide a strong support network and help combat feelings of loneliness.

Join a club or organization: Consider joining a club or organization that aligns with your interests, such as a book club, gardening group, or fitness class. This can be a great way to meet new people, stay active, and engage in activities that bring you joy.

Volunteer in your community: Volunteering is a wonderful way to give back to your community and make a positive impact. Whether it's helping out at a local food bank, mentoring a young person, or participating in a community clean-up event, volunteering can provide a sense of purpose and connection to others.

Attend community events: Keep an eye out for local events and activities happening in your community, such as farmers markets, concerts, or cultural festivals. Attending these events can help you stay connected to your community and engage in new experiences.

Take a class or workshop: Consider enrolling in a class or workshop to learn something new or develop a new skill. Whether it's painting, cooking, or learning a new language, taking a class can provide a fun and stimulating way to connect with others and stay engaged.

Stay active online: In today's digital age, social connections can also be maintained through online platforms. Consider joining social media groups, online forums, or virtual clubs to connect with others who share your interests.

By staying connected and involved in our communities, we can continue to lead fulfilling and meaningful lives as we age. Social connections and community involvement play a vital role in our overall well-being, providing support, companionship, and a sense of belonging. So take the time to nurture your relationships, explore new opportunities for engagement, and stay connected to the world around you. Your future self will thank you for it.

Chapter 7: The Importance of Sleep for Active Aging

Sleep is a fundamental aspect of our health that becomes even more crucial as we age. Quality sleep is essential for maintaining overall well-being, especially for active aging individuals. In this chapter, we will explore the importance of sleep for active aging and discuss strategies to improve sleep quality and duration for better overall health.

The Importance of Sleep for Active Aging

Quality sleep plays a vital role in maintaining physical, mental, and emotional health. As we age, our sleep patterns often change, with many older adults experiencing difficulty falling asleep, staying asleep, or achieving restful sleep. This can have a significant impact on overall health and quality of life.

Research has shown that inadequate sleep can contribute to a variety of health issues, including increased risk of chronic conditions such as heart disease, diabetes, and obesity. Poor sleep can also impair cognitive function, memory, and decision-making abilities, making it more challenging to engage in daily activities and maintain independence as we age.

For active aging individuals, quality sleep is particularly important for maintaining energy levels, supporting physical activity, and promoting recovery from exercise. A good night's sleep can help improve physical performance, reduce the risk of injury, and enhance overall well-being.

How to Improve Sleep Quality and Duration for Better Overall Health

Fortunately, there are several strategies that active aging individuals can implement to improve sleep quality and duration. These include:

Establish a bedtime routine: Developing a consistent bedtime routine can help signal to your body that it is time to wind down and prepare for sleep. This may include activities such as reading, listening to calming music, or practicing relaxation techniques.

Create a sleep-friendly environment: Ensure that your bedroom is a comfortable and relaxing space conducive to sleep. This may involve adjusting the temperature, minimizing noise and light, and investing in a comfortable mattress and pillows.

Limit screen time before bed: The blue light emitted by electronic devices such as smartphones, tablets, and computers can disrupt the production of melatonin, a hormone that regulates sleep-wake cycles. Limiting screen time before bed can help promote better sleep.

Stay active during the day: Engaging in regular physical activity can help improve sleep quality and duration.

Aim for at least 150 minutes of moderate-intensity exercise per week, such as walking, cycling, or swimming.

Practice good sleep hygiene: Incorporate habits that promote good sleep hygiene, such as avoiding caffeine and heavy meals close to bedtime, establishing a regular sleep schedule, and creating a relaxing bedtime routine.

Seek professional help if needed: If you continue to experience sleep difficulties despite implementing these strategies, consider seeking help from a healthcare provider or sleep specialist. They can help identify any underlying sleep disorders and develop a treatment plan tailored to your needs.

By prioritizing quality sleep, active aging individuals can support their overall health and well-being, enabling them to continue engaging in the activities they enjoy and maintaining independence as they age.

Incorporating these strategies into your daily routine can help improve sleep quality and duration, ultimately contributing to a healthier and more active lifestyle.

As we age, our bodies undergo various changes that can increase our risk of developing chronic conditions. However, by making healthy lifestyle choices, we can prevent and manage many common age-related health conditions. In this chapter, we will discuss tips for managing chronic conditions through lifestyle changes.

One of the most important steps in preventing and managing chronic conditions is maintaining a healthy diet. A diet rich in fruits, vegetables, whole grains, and lean protein can help reduce the risk of developing conditions such as heart disease, diabetes, and high blood pressure. It is also important to limit the intake of processed foods, sugary drinks, and foods high in saturated fats, as these can contribute to the development of chronic conditions.

Regular physical activity is another key component of preventing and managing chronic conditions. Exercise has been shown to improve cardiovascular health, reduce the risk of diabetes, and help maintain a healthy weight. Aim for at least 150 minutes of moderate-intensity exercise each week, such as brisk walking, swimming, or cycling. Strength training exercises, such as lifting weights or using resistance bands, can also help improve muscle strength and flexibility.

In addition to diet and exercise, managing stress is crucial for preventing and managing chronic conditions. Chronic stress can contribute to the development of conditions such as heart disease, depression, and anxiety. To reduce stress, try incorporating relaxation techniques into your daily routine, such as deep breathing, meditation, or yoga. Engaging in activities you enjoy, spending time with loved ones, and getting an adequate amount of sleep can also help reduce stress levels.

Another important aspect of preventing and managing chronic conditions is getting regular check-ups and screenings. Regular visits to your healthcare provider can help detect conditions early, when they are easier to treat. Make sure to follow your healthcare provider's recommendations for screenings, such as blood pressure checks, cholesterol tests, and mammograms or colonoscopies.

It is also important to take medications as prescribed by your healthcare provider. Skipping doses or stopping medications prematurely can worsen chronic conditions and lead to complications. If you experience any side effects or have concerns about your medications, be sure to discuss them with your healthcare provider.

In addition to these lifestyle changes, there are specific tips for managing common age-related health conditions:

Heart disease: To prevent heart disease, focus on maintaining a healthy weight, eating a balanced diet, exercising regularly, and managing stress. If you have been diagnosed with heart disease, follow your healthcare provider's recommendations for medications, lifestyle changes, and monitoring your condition.

Diabetes: If you have diabetes, it is important to monitor your blood sugar levels regularly, eat a balanced diet, exercise regularly, and take medications as prescribed. Work with your healthcare provider to create a diabetes management plan that works for you.

Arthritis: Managing arthritis involves staying active, maintaining a healthy weight, and protecting your joints. Low-impact exercises, such as swimming or tai chi, can help improve joint flexibility and reduce pain. Using assistive devices, such as braces or splints, can also help support your joints.

Osteoporosis: To prevent osteoporosis, focus on getting an adequate amount of calcium and vitamin D through your diet or supplements. Weight-bearing exercises, such as walking or dancing, can help strengthen bones and reduce the risk of fractures. If you have been diagnosed with osteoporosis, follow your healthcare provider's recommendations for medications and lifestyle changes.

By making healthy lifestyle choices, staying active, managing stress, and following your healthcare provider's recommendations, you can prevent and manage many common age-related health conditions. Remember that it is never too late to start making positive changes for your health.

Chapter 9: Balancing Work and Leisure in Retirement

Retirement is often viewed as a time for relaxation and leisure, a well-deserved break from the rigors of the working world. However, for many retirees, the transition from a busy career to a more leisurely lifestyle can be challenging. Some retirees find themselves feeling lost or unfulfilled without the structure and purpose that work provides. Others struggle to find a balance between work, leisure, and relaxation in retirement.

Finding the right balance between work and leisure in retirement is essential for maintaining a sense of fulfillment and satisfaction in this new chapter of life. Here are some tips and advice on how to achieve a fulfilling balance in retirement:

Assess Your Interests and Passions: Take some time to reflect on what activities and pursuits bring you joy and fulfillment. Consider your hobbies, interests, and values, and think about how you can incorporate these into your retirement lifestyle. Whether it's volunteering, pursuing a new hobby, or starting a small business, finding activities that align with your passions can help you stay engaged and fulfilled in retirement.

Set Goals and Prioritize Your Time: Just as you did in your career, it's important to set goals and prioritize your time in retirement. Determine what activities are most important to you and allocate your time accordingly. Whether it's spending time with family and friends, pursuing a new hobby, or taking on part-time work, setting goals can help you stay focused and motivated in retirement.

Embrace a Flexible Schedule: One of the benefits of retirement is the freedom to create your own schedule. Embrace this flexibility and allow yourself to adjust your routine as needed. Be open to trying new activities and experiences, and don't be afraid to change course if something isn't working for you. A flexible schedule can help you find a balance between work, leisure, and relaxation in retirement.

Find Meaningful Work: For some retirees, work is an important source of fulfillment and purpose. If you find that you miss the structure and sense of accomplishment that work provided, consider finding meaningful work in retirement. This could be part-time work, volunteering, or starting a small business. Finding work that aligns with your interests and values can help you stay engaged and fulfilled in retirement.

Practice Self-Care: In the midst of balancing work and leisure in retirement, it's important to prioritize self-care.

Make time for activities that help you relax and recharge, such as exercise, meditation, or spending time outdoors. Taking care of your physical, emotional, and mental well-being is essential for maintaining a fulfilling and healthy retirement lifestyle.

Seek Support and Connection: Retirement can be a time of transition and adjustment, and it's important to seek support and connection during this period. Stay connected with family and friends, join social groups or clubs, or participate in community activities. Building a support network can help you navigate the challenges of retirement and find a balance between work, leisure, and relaxation.

Finding a fulfilling balance between work, leisure, and relaxation in retirement is a personal journey that will look different for each individual.

By assessing your interests and passions, setting goals, embracing a flexible schedule, finding meaningful work, practicing self-care, and seeking support and connection, you can create a retirement lifestyle that is fulfilling, rewarding, and balanced. Embrace this new chapter of life with enthusiasm and openness, and remember that retirement is a time for exploration, growth, and self-discovery.

Chapter 10: Embracing Technology for Active Aging

As we age, it is important to stay active and engaged in order to maintain our physical and mental well-being. Technology has become an essential tool in helping us achieve this goal, providing us with countless resources and opportunities to enhance our active aging journey. In this chapter, we will explore how to leverage technology to support and empower ourselves as we age gracefully.

One of the key benefits of technology for active aging is the ability to track and monitor our health and fitness goals. There are a wide range of wearable devices and mobile apps available that can help us stay on track with our exercise routine, monitor our heart rate and sleep patterns, and even remind us to take our medications. By using these tools, we can better understand our health trends and make informed decisions about how to improve our overall well-being.

In addition to monitoring our physical health, technology can also support our mental and emotional well-being. Social media platforms and online communities provide us with opportunities to connect with others who share similar interests and experiences, reducing feelings of isolation and loneliness. Video calling services, such as Skype and FaceTime, allow us to stay in touch with family and friends, even if they are miles away. These tools can help us maintain strong social connections and support networks as we age.

Another benefit of technology for active aging is the access to educational resources and opportunities for lifelong learning. Online courses and webinars offer us the chance to explore new subjects and interests, keeping our minds sharp and engaged. E-books and audiobooks make it easier for us to access a wealth of information and literature, regardless of our physical limitations or mobility challenges.

By embracing technology as a learning tool, we can continue to expand our knowledge and pursue our passions well into our golden years.

Furthermore, technology can simplify our daily tasks and routines, making it easier for us to maintain our independence and autonomy as we age. Smart home devices, such as voice-activated assistants and automated lighting systems, can help us manage our household chores and stay safe in our own homes. Online shopping services and delivery apps allow us to access groceries, medications, and other essentials without leaving the comfort of our home. By leveraging these tools, we can maintain our quality of life and age in place with dignity and grace.

As we embrace technology for active aging, it is important to stay informed and educated about the latest trends and developments in the digital world. Attend workshops and seminars on technology for seniors, read articles and blogs on aging and technology, and seek guidance from tech-savvy friends and family members.

By staying proactive and curious, we can stay ahead of the curve and make the most of the technological tools available to us.

In conclusion, technology has the power to enhance our active aging journey in countless ways. By leveraging wearable devices, mobile apps, social media platforms, online learning resources, and smart home devices, we can stay connected, engaged, and independent as we age gracefully. Embrace technology as a valuable ally in your active aging journey, and reap the benefits of a healthier, happier, and more fulfilling life.

Chapter 11: Travel and Adventure in Later Life

As we age, it is common for many individuals to start thinking about how they want to spend their retirement years. For some, this may involve embarking on new adventures and exploring different parts of the world. Travel and adventure in later life can be an exciting and fulfilling experience, but it also requires careful planning and consideration. In this chapter, we will discuss some tips for planning and enjoying travel adventures in later life.

One of the first things to consider when planning a travel adventure in later life is the destination. It is important to choose a destination that is both appealing and suitable for your individual needs and preferences. Consider factors such as climate, accessibility, and activities available in the area. Additionally, it may be helpful to consult with a travel agent or do some research online to find destinations that cater to older adults and offer amenities such as accessible accommodations and transportation options.

Once you have chosen a destination, it is important to plan your trip carefully. Make sure to research local customs, attractions, and transportation options in advance. Consider any health concerns or mobility limitations you may have and plan accordingly. It may be helpful to create a detailed itinerary and make reservations for accommodations and activities ahead of time to ensure a smooth and stress-free travel experience.

When traveling in later life, it is important to prioritize your health and safety. Make sure to pack any necessary medications, medical supplies, and travel insurance. Stay hydrated, eat well, and get plenty of rest to avoid fatigue and illness while traveling. It may also be helpful to bring along a list of emergency contacts and important medical information in case of an emergency.

While traveling in later life, it is important to pace yourself and take breaks as needed. Consider scheduling rest days or shorter excursions to prevent exhaustion and allow time for relaxation. Listen to your body and do not push yourself beyond your limits. Remember, the goal of travel and adventure in later life is to enjoy new experiences and create lasting memories, so take the time to savor each moment and appreciate the journey.

Another important aspect of travel and adventure in later life is staying connected with loved ones. Make sure to share your travel plans with family and friends and check in regularly to let them know you are safe and enjoying your trip. Consider bringing along a phone or other communication device to stay in touch while traveling. Additionally, consider documenting your adventures through photos, journals, or social media to share with others and preserve your memories for years to come.

In conclusion, travel and adventure in later life can be a rewarding and enriching experience, but it requires careful planning and consideration. By choosing a suitable destination, planning your trip carefully, prioritizing your health and safety, pacing yourself, staying connected with loved ones, and savoring each moment, you can enjoy a fulfilling and memorable travel adventure in later life. Remember, age is just a number, and it is never too late to explore the world and embark on new adventures. So pack your bags, hit the road, and make the most of your golden years with travel and adventure.

Chapter 12: Cultivating a Positive Mindset

Having a positive mindset is crucial for navigating life's challenges with grace and resilience. It is the foundation upon which we can build a fulfilling and meaningful life. Cultivating a positive mindset is not always easy, especially when faced with adversity or setbacks. However, with the right strategies and practices, it is possible to maintain a positive outlook and bounce back from even the most difficult situations.

One of the key strategies for cultivating a positive mindset is practicing gratitude. Gratitude is the practice of acknowledging and appreciating the good things in your life, no matter how small. By focusing on the positive aspects of your life, you can shift your perspective from one of lack and negativity to one of abundance and positivity. Keeping a gratitude journal, where you write down things you are grateful for each day, can be a powerful tool for cultivating a positive mindset.

Another important strategy for maintaining a positive outlook is practicing mindfulness. Mindfulness is the practice of being fully present in the moment, without judgment. By learning to stay present and aware of your thoughts and emotions, you can cultivate a sense of calm and peace, even in the midst of chaos. Mindfulness can help you let go of negative thoughts and emotions, and cultivate a more positive and optimistic outlook on life.

In addition to gratitude and mindfulness, it is important to practice self-care in order to cultivate a positive mindset. Self-care involves taking care of your physical, emotional, and mental well-being. This can include things like getting enough sleep, eating nutritious foods, exercising regularly, and engaging in activities that bring you joy and relaxation. Taking care of yourself is essential for maintaining a positive mindset and building resilience in the face of challenges.

Another strategy for cultivating a positive mindset is to cultivate a growth mindset. A growth mindset is the belief that our abilities and intelligence can be developed through hard work, effort, and perseverance. By adopting a growth mindset, you can view challenges as opportunities for growth and learning, rather than obstacles to be avoided. This can help you stay positive and motivated, even when faced with setbacks or failures.

Finally, it is important to surround yourself with positive and supportive people in order to cultivate a positive mindset. The people you surround yourself with can have a big impact on your outlook on life. Surrounding yourself with positive, uplifting people who believe in you and support you can help you stay positive and resilient in the face of challenges. Conversely, being around negative, toxic people can drain your energy and dampen your spirits. Choose your relationships wisely and cultivate a supportive network of friends and family who uplift and inspire you.

In conclusion, cultivating a positive mindset is essential for navigating life's challenges with resilience and grace. By practicing gratitude, mindfulness, self-care, adopting a growth mindset, and surrounding yourself with positive and supportive people, you can cultivate a positive outlook on life and build the resilience needed to overcome even the most difficult situations. Remember that positivity is a choice, and with the right strategies and practices, you can cultivate a positive mindset that will serve you well in all areas of your life.

Conclusion: Your Youthful You Journey

As you reach the end of your Youthful You journey, it is important to take a moment to reflect on all that you have accomplished and celebrate the achievements you have made along the way. This program was designed to help you embrace active aging and live your life to the fullest, and it is clear that you have done just that.

Throughout this journey, you have challenged yourself in ways you never thought possible. Whether it was trying a new exercise routine, learning a new hobby, or pushing yourself outside of your comfort zone, you have shown incredible determination and perseverance. You have proven that age is just a number and that it is never too late to make positive changes in your life.

But the Youthful You journey was not just about physical activity – it was also about nourishing your mind and soul.

You have engaged in activities that have sparked your creativity, stimulated your intellect, and fostered personal growth. You have cultivated meaningful relationships, explored new interests, and discovered what truly brings you joy and fulfillment.

As you reflect on your journey, take time to celebrate all that you have achieved. Celebrate the strength and resilience you have demonstrated in the face of challenges. Celebrate the new skills and knowledge you have acquired. Celebrate the friendships you have formed and the memories you have created. Celebrate the positive changes you have made in your life and the impact they have had on your overall well-being.

But remember, the Youthful You journey does not have to end here. This program was designed to be a springboard for continued growth and exploration. As you move forward, continue to challenge yourself, learn new things, and seek out opportunities for personal development.

Embrace change and embrace the journey of active aging with open arms.

In conclusion, your Youthful You journey has been a testament to your strength, determination, and resilience. You have taken control of your life and embraced the power of active aging, and the results speak for themselves. As you continue on your journey, remember to celebrate your achievements, reflect on your growth, and always strive to be the best version of yourself. Your journey is far from over – embrace it with enthusiasm and continue to live your life to the fullest.

Next Steps: Resources for Continued Active Aging

As we age, it is important to continue to prioritize our physical and mental well-being in order to maintain an active and healthy lifestyle. In this chapter, we will explore various resources and support systems that can help older adults stay engaged, active, and independent as they age.

Community Centers and Senior Centers Community centers and senior centers offer a wide range of programs and activities specifically designed for older adults. These can include exercise classes, art workshops, social events, educational seminars, and much more. These centers provide a supportive environment for older adults to stay active and engaged with their community.

Fitness and Wellness Programs Many gyms and fitness centers offer specialized programs for older adults, such as senior fitness classes, water aerobics, yoga, and Tai Chi.

These programs are designed to improve strength, flexibility, balance, and overall physical health. Additionally, many communities have walking clubs and hiking groups that provide opportunities for older adults to stay active outdoors.

Volunteer Opportunities Volunteering is a great way for older adults to stay engaged with their community and make a positive impact. There are numerous organizations that rely on volunteers, such as food banks, animal shelters, hospitals, schools, and environmental groups. Volunteering can provide a sense of purpose and fulfillment, as well as opportunities for social interaction and physical activity.

Continuing Education Many colleges and universities offer continuing education programs specifically for older adults. These programs cover a wide range of topics, such as art, history, literature, technology, and language.

Continuing education classes can stimulate the mind, promote lifelong learning, and provide opportunities for social interaction with peers.

Support Groups Support groups can be a valuable resource for older adults who are facing specific challenges or health issues. There are support groups for individuals with chronic conditions, caregivers, grief and loss, and many other topics. These groups provide a safe space for individuals to share their experiences, receive emotional support, and learn coping strategies.

Technology Resources Technology can be a powerful tool for older adults to stay connected with loved ones, access information, and engage in activities. Many older adults benefit from using smartphones, tablets, and computers to stay in touch with family and friends, participate in virtual social events, and access online resources. There are also numerous apps and websites specifically designed for older adults to promote cognitive health and physical fitness.

Transportation Services Access to reliable transportation is essential for older adults to maintain their independence and stay engaged in their community. Many communities offer transportation services specifically for older adults, such as paratransit, senior shuttles, and volunteer driver programs. Additionally, ride-sharing services and taxis can provide convenient options for getting around town.

Home Care Services For older adults who may need assistance with daily tasks, such as cooking, cleaning, and personal care, home care services can provide the support they need to continue living independently. Home care services can be tailored to individual needs and preferences, and can help older adults maintain their health and well-being in the comfort of their own homes.

By utilizing these resources and support systems, older adults can continue to lead active, fulfilling, and independent lives as they age. It is important to explore the options available in your community and find the resources that best fit your needs and interests.

 Remember that staying active and engaged is a lifelong journey, and there are always opportunities for growth and enrichment at every stage of life.

Notes

Notes

Notes

Thank You For Your Support

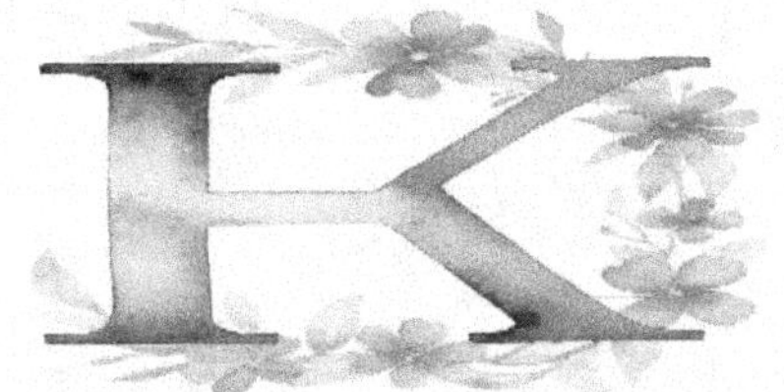